SURGICAL TECHNOLOGY STUDENTS
ARE YOU READY FOR THE CLINICAL ROTATION?

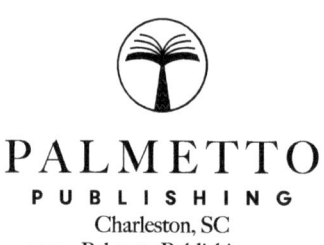

PALMETTO
PUBLISHING
Charleston, SC
www.PalmettoPublishing.com

Copyright © 2024 by Francisca Soetan, EdD, CST

All rights reserved

No portion of this book may be reproduced, stored in a retrieval system, or transmitted in any form by any means–electronic, mechanical, photocopy, recording, or other–except for brief quotations in printed reviews, without prior permission of the author.

Hardcover ISBN: 9798822962941
Paperback ISBN: 9798822962958
eBook ISBN: 9798822962965

SURGICAL TECHNOLOGY STUDENTS

ARE YOU READY FOR THE CLINICAL ROTATION?

Clinical Rotation Guide for
The Surgical Technology Student

A Handbook for Surgical Technology
Clinical Rotation First Edition

BASED ON AST Core Curriculum for
Surgical Technology Seventh Edition

FRANCISCA SOETAN, EdD, CST

To all Surgical Technology Instructors.
Thank you for teaching and for ensuring the safety
of surgical patients.

Bisola, Moriam and Feyisola, thank you for your support.

TABLE OF CONTENTS

Introduction 1
For Medical Clearance 2
Appearance. 4
Code of Ethics Agreement Contract. 8
First Day On-Site and Daily Attendance 10
    First Day. 10
    Attendance and Absences. 13
    Unacceptable Behaviors 13
(HIPAA) Health Insurance Portability and Accountability Act of 1996. 16
Real-life Situation 18
    Instrument Count 18
    Patient's Safety 20
    YOUR Safety 20
    Emergency Life Saving Activity. 22
    Surgical Conscience 22
Surgical Rotation Case Requirements 23
    General Surgery. 23
    Specialty surgery. 25
    Surgical Specialties (excluding General Surgery) . . . 27

Surgical Rotation Case and Role Documentation 29
    Hit the Ground Running 29
    Case Recording Tools:. 33

Assignments 35
    A Learning and Practice Tool: Case Notes. 35
    Surgical Case Report. 39
    Continuing Education Articles 44

Basic MLA Format 45

Manual Surgical Case Recording Tool 48

    General surgery. 48
    Observation role 49
    Cardiothoracic. 50
    Genitourinary. 50
    Neurology. 51
    Obstetrics and Gynecology. 51
    Orthopedic. 52
    Otorhinolaryngology 52
    Ophthalmology 53
    Oral Maxillofacial 53
    Peripheral vascular 54
    Plastics and reconstructive 54
    Procurement and transplant 55
    Endoscopy 55
    Notes. 56

About the Author. 60

INTRODUCTION

Congratulations! You made it past the preliminary level. Now, it's time for your hands-on training. Clinical rotations are simply the time that you spend in a hospital to gain real-life experience in real operating rooms and, most importantly, with real patients, not mannequins. During these periods, as a student learner, you will gain experience by assisting surgeons working with patients and performing surgical procedures in real hospital settings. Clinical rotation is a crucial study that you must complete to be eligible for graduation and the certification exam and to eventually become the surgical tech you aspire to be.

Yay!

When it comes to your clinical rotation, it is important to know what to expect, what you should do, what you should not do, and the expectations of your college and the clinical sites. It is crucial to understand that clinical rotations are not paid jobs or internships. You are not considered an employee at the clinical sites.

Let us carefully go over some important information before embarking on that sweet journey of finally stepping into the real operating room.

SURGICAL TECHNOLOGY STUDENTS

FOR MEDICAL CLEARANCE

a. You are required to undergo a physical examination conducted by your physician.

b. You must comply with all vaccine requirements.

c. You must agree to a drug screening.

d. The drug test must come back negative.

e. Mask fitting and other requirements by the hospital must be completed before your clinical start date.

f. Every hospital may have different protocols for processing clinical student applications, so be prepared to follow all protocols.

ARE YOU READY FOR THE CLINICAL ROTATION?

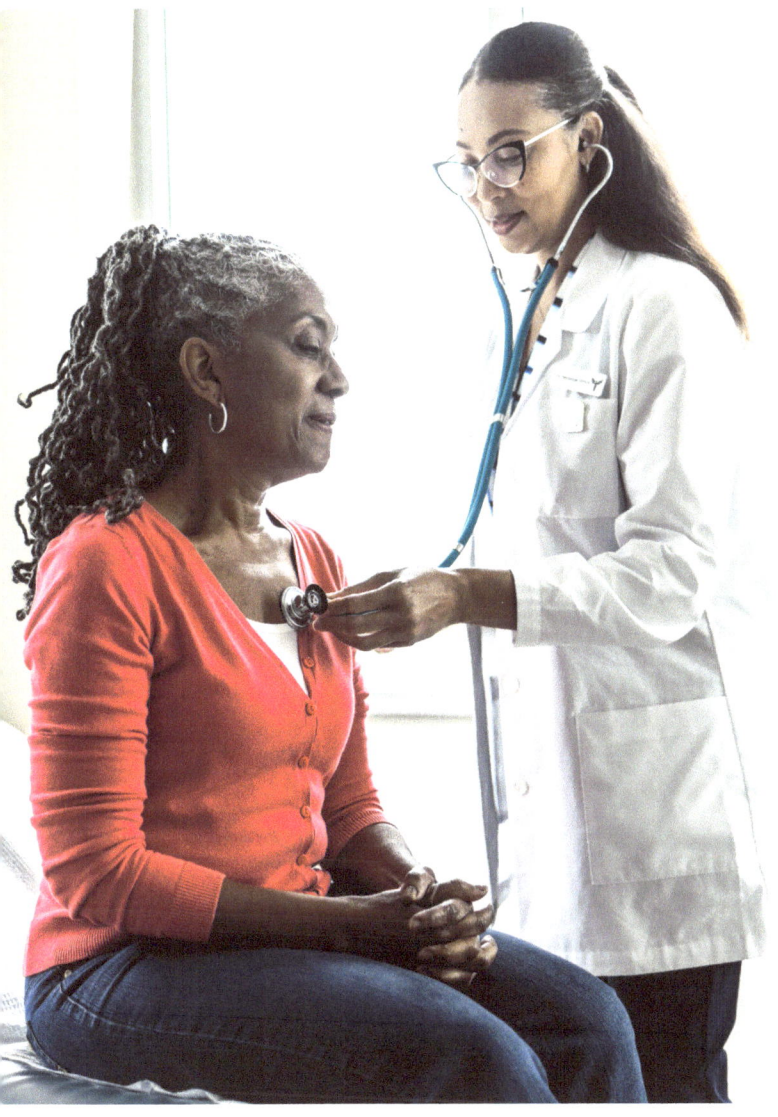

APPEARANCE

Nails and accessories that we wear daily may contain bacteria. Our appearance in the Operating Room (OR) and/or what we wear may unintentionally become sources of bacterial infection for patients in the OR. These bacterial infections may turn deadly. To avoid the chance of infection, there are some strict rules that we must adhere to before going into the OR and participating in any surgical procedure. Some hospitals may have other rules for you to follow, so please follow all rules as required by the specific hospital and OR. Here are a few definite rules and tips that you must remember:

a. No long nails allowed. (Nails must be cut to the nail bed).

b. No artificial nails or nail polish. Although some hospitals allow their surgical technologists to wear fresh nail polish with no sign of chipping in the operating room, you, as a student, are not allowed to wear any nail polish at all.

c. You must change into hospital-laundered scrubs when you arrive at the hospital during your clinical hours. (You will be given access to the scrub machine or paper scrubs).

d. If you need to go to another department in the hospital, you must wear a lab coat over your scrubs. The lab coats will be provided to you in the OR or in the scrub machine. Most ORs have disposable lab coats available for your use. If you need to go outside of the hospital for any reason, ask your instructor for permission. Do not wear your hospital-assigned scrubs outside of the hospital. Take the scrubs off before going out of the hospital and don a fresh set from the machine as soon as you return.

e. Make sure your hairstyle can fit under the operating room bouffant hat. Your hair should not be visible or dangling from under the hat. For facial hair, there are facial hair covers available in the OR.

f. Avoid wearing any kind of perfume during your clinical hours. Some patients may be allergic to fragrances; therefore wearing them may cause serious allergic reactions.

g. No large or dangling earrings.

h. You should try to eat breakfast in the morning to enhance stamina and concentration.

i. You may bring beverages and snacks to eat during long or short breaks.

j. Very important: there is no eating allowed in the OR. You must leave all snacks in your locker and eat in the breakroom, locker room, or another area designated for eating.

k. Do not bring food or snacks into the OR.

l. You must take all hand jewelry off before going into the OR. Yes, this includes your wedding band.

m. Dangling neckwear must be removed or tucked inside your scrub top, and you must tuck in your scrub top before you start scrubbing. Dangling neckwear can cause contamination if it dangles over your sterile field.

n. All cell phones must be turned off when entering the operating room. It's best to keep your turned-off cell phone in your scrubs pocket.

o. Until personal lockers are assigned, please avoid bringing valuables to the hospital, as you may need a locker to store them.

ARE YOU READY FOR THE CLINICAL ROTATION?

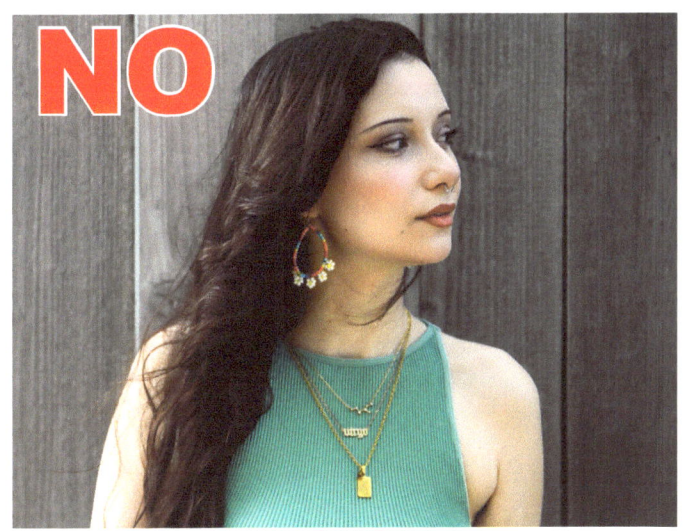

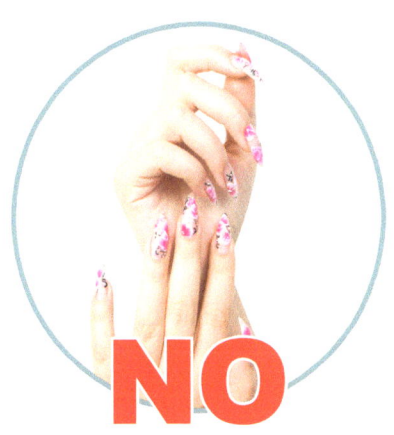

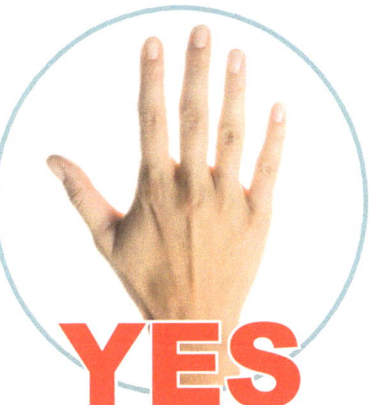

SURGICAL TECHNOLOGY STUDENTS

CODE OF ETHICS AGREEMENT CONTRACT

Students are expected to follow the code of ethics in the hospitals they are assigned to and agree to be responsible for their actions. You will be required to sign an ethical agreement contract agreeing to follow rules of conduct which include but are not limited to:

- Responsibility for Patient Care
- Respect for Persons
- Respect for Patient Confidentiality (remember HIPAA!)
- Honesty and Integrity
- Professional Behavior
- Conscientiousness

ARE YOU READY FOR THE CLINICAL ROTATION?

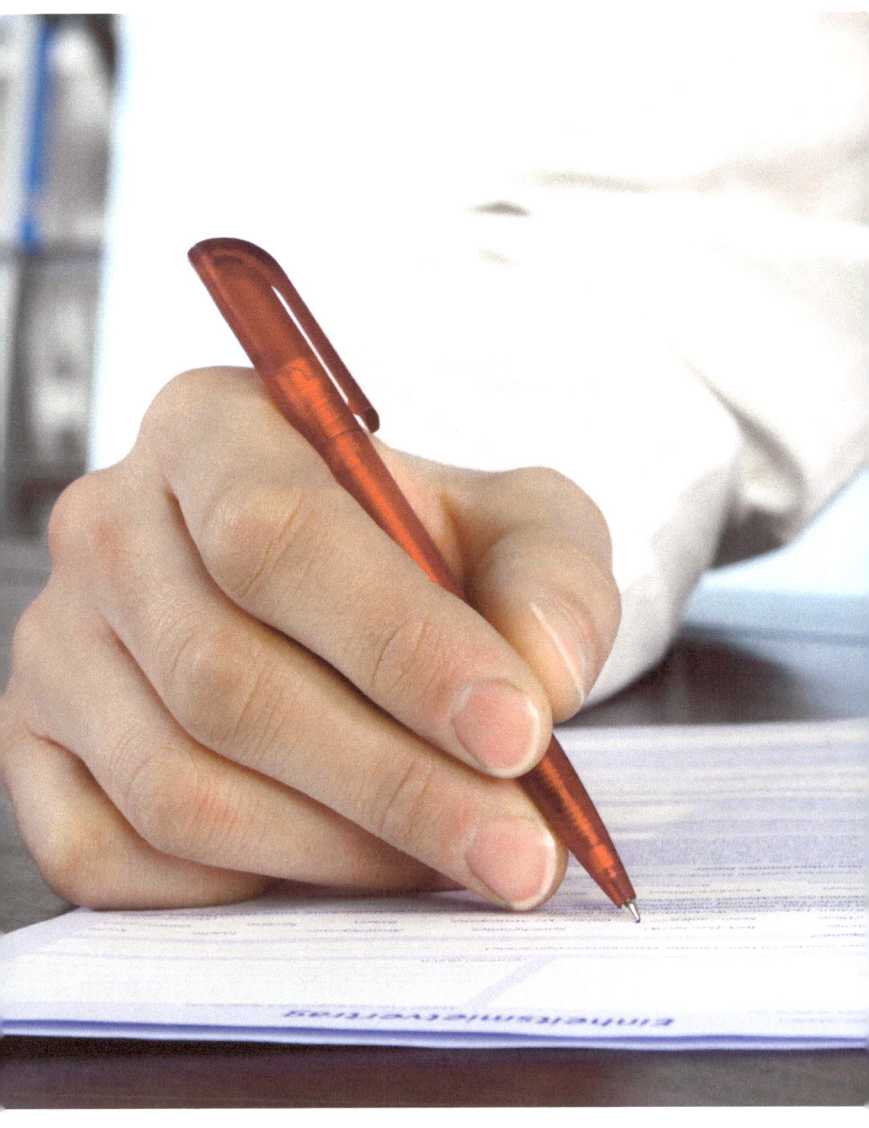

FIRST DAY ON-SITE AND DAILY ATTENDANCE

FIRST DAY

You are expected to meet with your clinical instructor at a designated area of the hospital. Most of the time, the lobby is the first place of meeting since you will need to meet at a common area of the hospital before proceeding to the office. Once at the office, you will be introduced to the OR nurse manager and directed to the appropriate department for your ID and scrub machine card. Very important: you must change into hospital scrubs during your clinical hours.

You will be introduced to your preceptors; these are the surgical technologists working in the hospital. The preceptors will be your teachers during clinical hours and will give a report on your performance to your clinical instructors at the end of the day. Although your clinical instructors may check on you in the room occasionally, the instructors rely on the preceptors' reports about your performance in the OR. Remember, the Staff Surgical Technologist is your preceptor. They are the only surgical team members to teach you the skills of surgical technology.

Although you will be introduced to the operating room staff on the first day of the clinical, you must introduce yourself every day as you step into the operating room. Do not just assume they already know you. Always treat each day as a first day by introducing yourself in the OR, especially to the surgeons. For example: "Good morning, Dr. Cutter. My name is Shine, and I am a student in the Shining Star surgical technology program. Thank you for the opportunity to learn." All hospitals have different protocols governing students in their facilities; therefore, be sure to follow all rules and regulations of the hospital at which you are placed for your clinical rotation.

If anything unusual happens in the operating room during your clinical hours, please bring it to the attention of your clinical instructor. Do not take any action on your own. If you are injured in the operating room for any reason, you must notify your instructor immediately. Your instructor will make proper arrangements to notify the school and ensure that all necessary protocols are followed. In the hospital, you will be required to fill out an incident report, which will be signed by the nurse supervisor or whomever is assigned by the hospital to oversee incident reports in the OR. Rest assured that all necessary steps will be taken to ensure that you are taken care of appropriately.

SURGICAL TECHNOLOGY STUDENTS

ATTENDANCE AND ABSENCES

Most operating rooms start very early, some as early as 5:00 a.m. Depending on your assigned clinical site, if you are required to get to your clinical site at 5:00 a.m., be prepared to get to the clinical site and don the OR attire by 5:00 a.m. No late arrival will be allowed. Absences should be kept to the minimum accepted by the program. If you are late numerous times, it may count as days of absences, depending on the hours of lateness accumulated. To be absent more than one day during the clinical rotation may end in a dismissal or a repeat of the class, depending on the situation. If your absence is excused, you may be allowed to repeat the class, but if your absence is not excused, you may be dismissed from the class and even the program entirely. We know that life happens; if your situation changes and affects your clinical hours due to family or other situations, your best bet is to contact your clinical instructor immediately. Your instructor will be able to advise you on possible options while in contact with the leadership of the department.

UNACCEPTABLE BEHAVIORS

Watch your language and attitude. The following are some of the behaviors and attitudes that you must not be found committing at your clinical site under any circumstances. They can result in immediate dismissal from the program:

- Use of foul language.
- Disrespect toward your instructor, hospital staff, patients, or fellow students.
- Physical or verbal altercation with your instructor, hospital staff, patient, or fellow student.
- Insubordination.
- Chronic lateness.

ARE YOU READY FOR THE CLINICAL ROTATION?

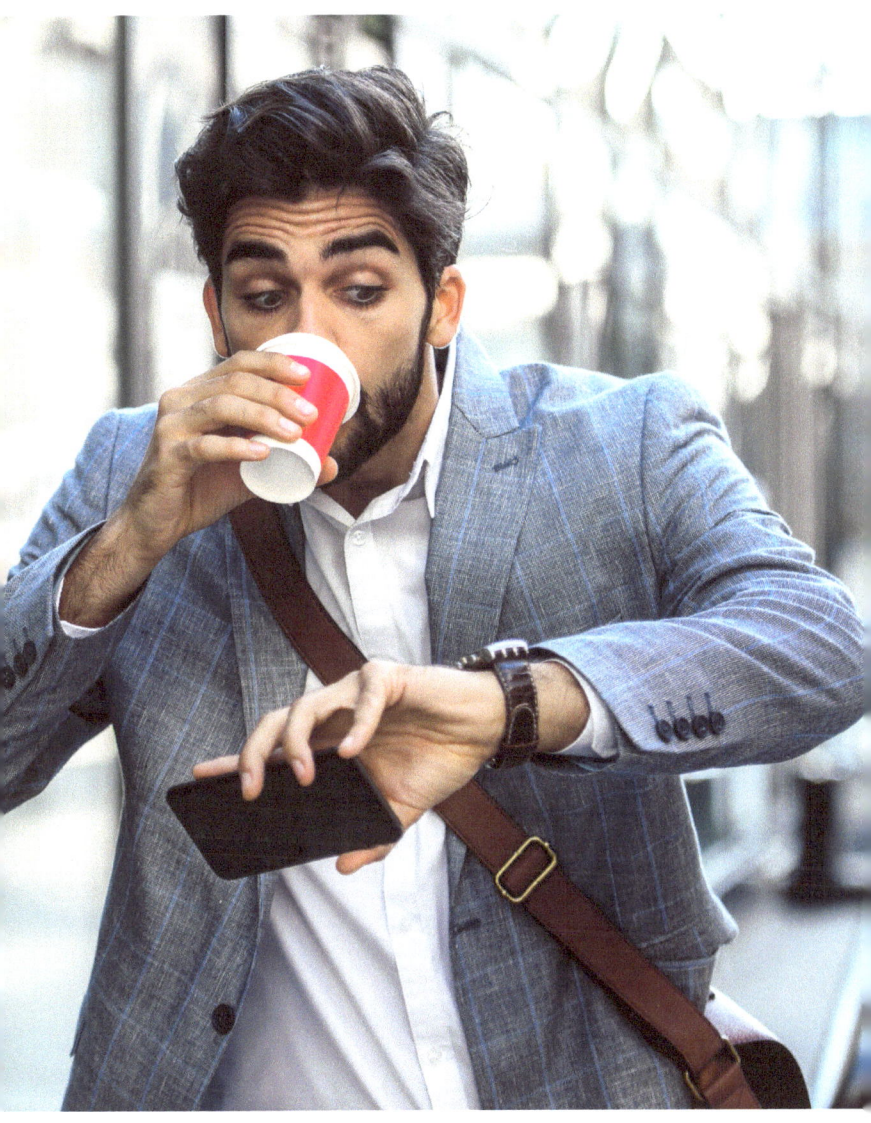

(HIPAA) HEALTH INSURANCE PORTABILITY AND ACCOUNTABILITY ACT OF 1996

The Health Insurance Portability and Accountability Act of 1996 (HIPAA) is a federal law that requires the creation of national standards to protect sensitive patient health information from being disclosed without the patient's consent or knowledge.

"Whatever happens in Vegas, stays in Vegas." Do not discuss your patients with anyone, even if you happen to see a neighbor or anyone that you know brought into the OR on a stretcher for an emergency procedure. Do not call any of the person's family members to inform them that their loved one is in the OR. Let the hospital handle the information according to the protocol. You are not to discuss any patient with your family members, friends, or coworkers. Violation of HIPAA may lead to termination of your clinical rotation and dismissal from the program.

ARE YOU READY FOR THE CLINICAL ROTATION?

REAL-LIFE SITUATION

Remember to "go with the flow." As real-life scenarios occur in the OR, you are not to argue with any of the surgical team members. Listen attentively and follow instructions and directives from the surgeon, the circulating nurse, the anesthesiologist, and your preceptor, the staff surgical technologist.

INSTRUMENT COUNT

You are required to count your instruments with the circulating nurse under the supervision of your preceptor before the case starts. However, if there is a surgical emergency, the instrument count may be suspended until the emergency is brought under control. The nurse will prompt you to count the instruments as soon as they see it makes sense to do so. Do not argue with the team about how you were taught in school that "the instruments are to be counted first." Remember, an emergency procedure must be embarked on as soon as the patient is wheeled into the operating suite. Only during emergencies can counting the instruments wait until the patient is stabilized. You simply need to keep track of your instruments as you hand them to the surgeon.

ARE YOU READY FOR THE CLINICAL ROTATION?

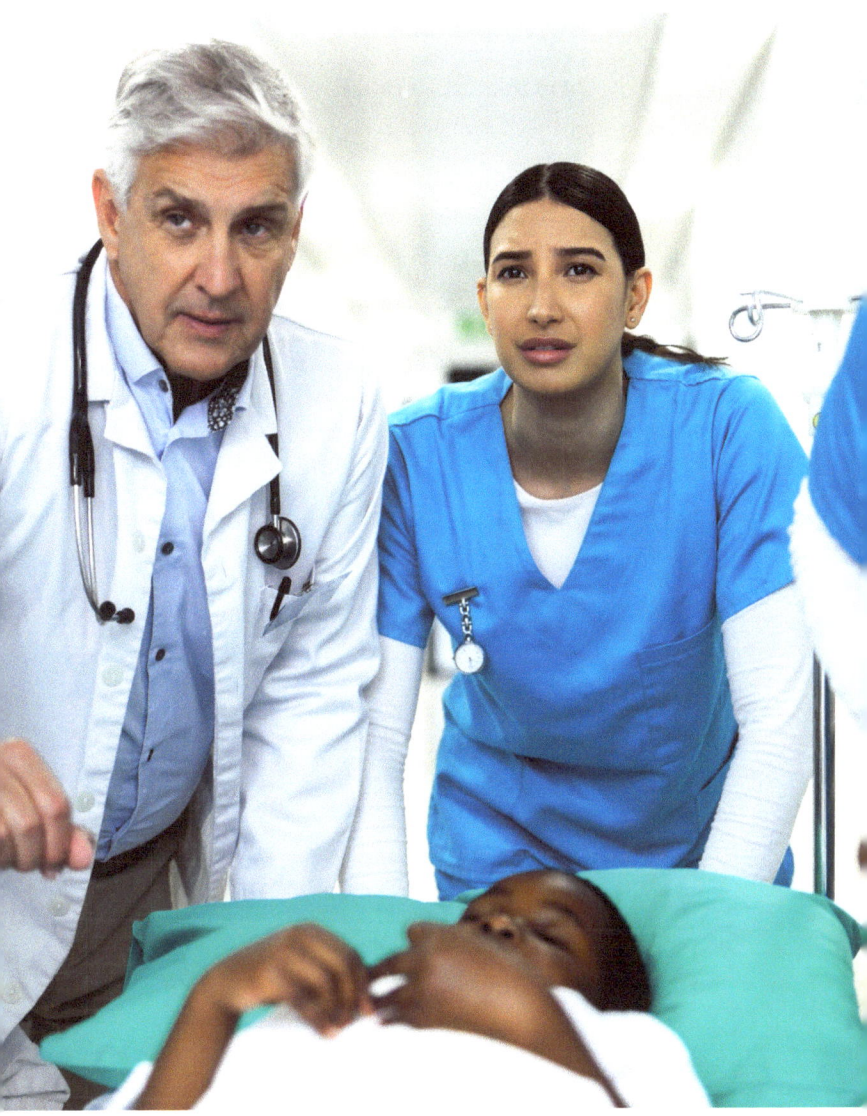

PATIENT'S SAFETY

You already know that after you are gowned and gloved in sterile PPE, you are not to touch any non-sterile surface; however, in the case of an emergency, you must take action. For example, you may notice a patient falling off the operating table before other team members have noticed. In this instance, it is important to take quick action by saving the patient from falling and calling the attention of the other team members to the situation. Your gown and gloves will be contaminated, but all you need is simply to return to the scrub sink to scrub and don sterile PPE once again. In this example, you saved a patient from serious injuries or even death. The sterile PPE can be replaced, but not the patient.

YOUR SAFETY

For your protection, always wear eye goggles whenever you scrub in <u>any</u> procedure. Do not get into the habit of "This is a small case; no need for eye goggles." Whenever you are in a room where an X-ray will be used, always wear a lead apron and a thyroid shield, regardless of your role, be it First Scrub, Second Scrub or Observation role. The hospital will provide lead aprons and thyroid shields.

ARE YOU READY FOR THE CLINICAL ROTATION?

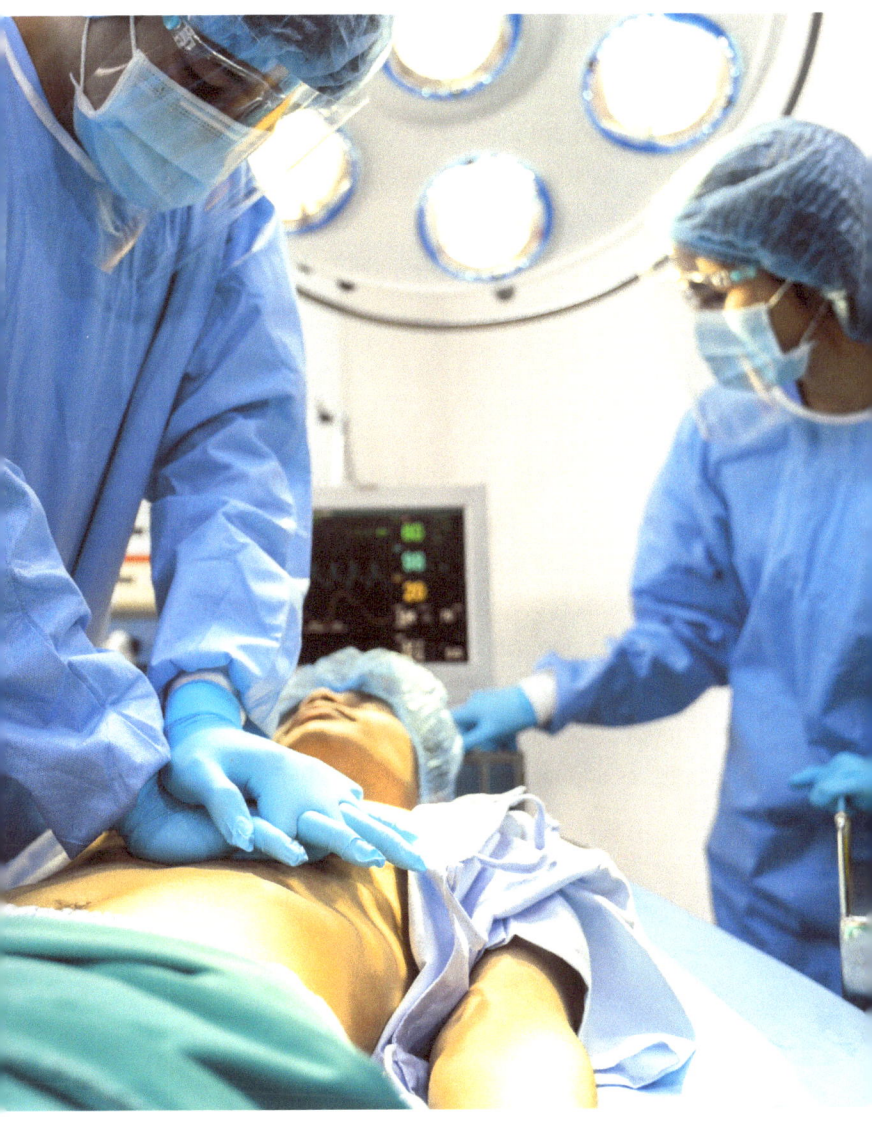

EMERGENCY LIFE SAVING ACTIVITY

Cardiac arrest may happen during a surgical procedure, which may require lifesaving acts like CPR and chest compressions. As long as you have pushed your backable and mayo stand aside and keep them sterile, you may participate in life saving compressions for a patient if you are requested to do so.

SURGICAL CONSCIENCE

As you were taught in the classroom and the school lab, one important action to take whenever there are questions about sterility is to address those questions and ensure that the situation is rectified by replacing any contaminated item with a sterile one. As a student, you are held to the same standard in the OR as the preceptor when it comes to contamination. You must uphold your knowledge of aseptic techniques and let your surgical conscience be guided by it.

SURGICAL ROTATION CASE REQUIREMENTS

Keywords and initialisms:
First Scrub Role (FS)
Second Scrub Role (SS)
Observation Role (O)

Case Requirements Breakdown According to AST Core Curriculum 7th Edition

Students must complete a minimum of **120 cases** as explained below:

GENERAL SURGERY

Students must complete a minimum of 30 cases of General Surgery.

- ✓ Of the 30 cases, 20 must be performed in the FS role.
- ✓ 10 cases of the 30 cases may be performed in the FS or SS role.

SURGICAL TECHNOLOGY STUDENTS

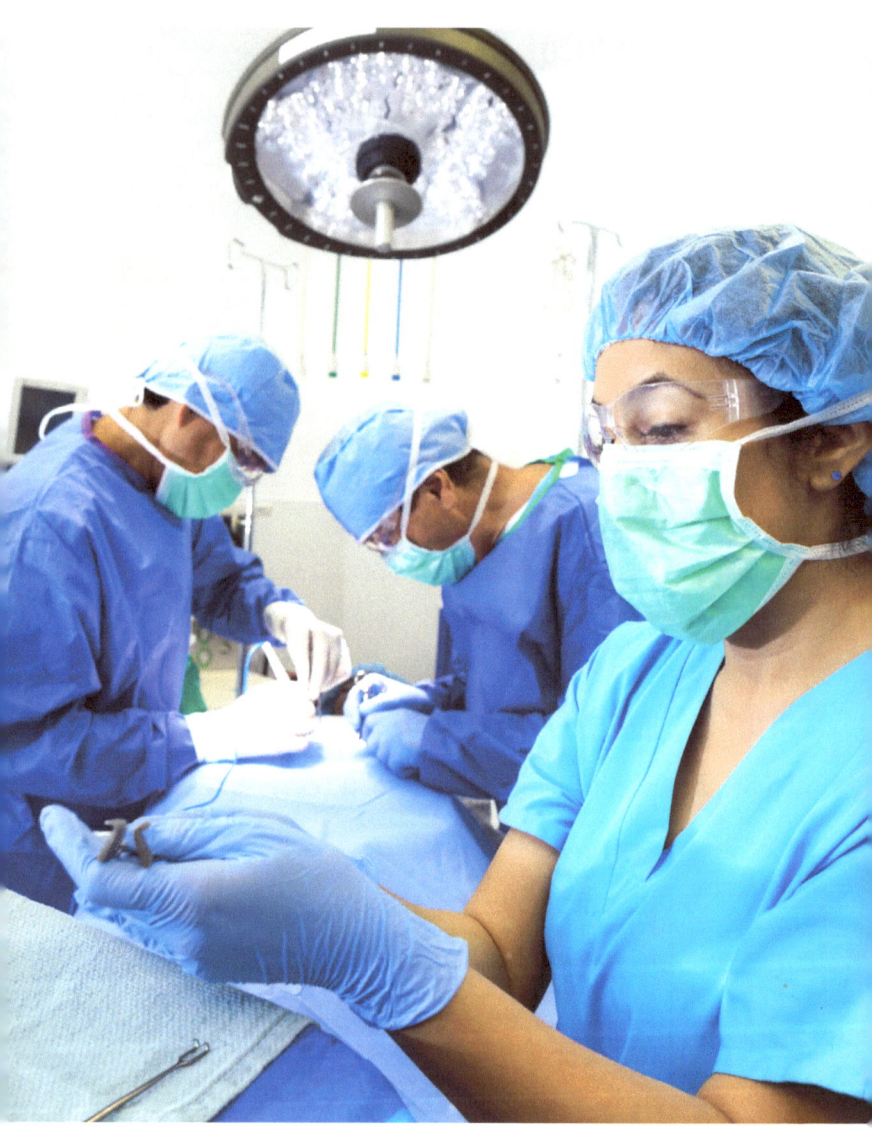

SPECIALTY SURGERY

Students must complete a minimum of **90 cases** in other surgical specialties, with a **minimum of 60 cases** performed in the **FS** role and distributed amongst a **minimum of FOUR surgical specialties**.

- ✓ A **minimum of ten cases in four different specialties** must be completed in the FS role (**total of 40**).
- ✓ The **additional 20 cases** in the FS role may be distributed amongst any one surgical specialty or multiple surgical specialties.
- ✓ The **remaining 30 cases** may be performed in any surgical specialty in either the FS or SS role.
- ✓ **A total of 10 endoscopy diagnostic** cases are counted in the **SS role**.
- ✓ A **total of FIVE** Vaginal delivery cases are counted in the SS role of the OB/GYN specialty.

SURGICAL CASE REQUIREMENTS DIAGRAM

AST Core Curriculum 7th Edition

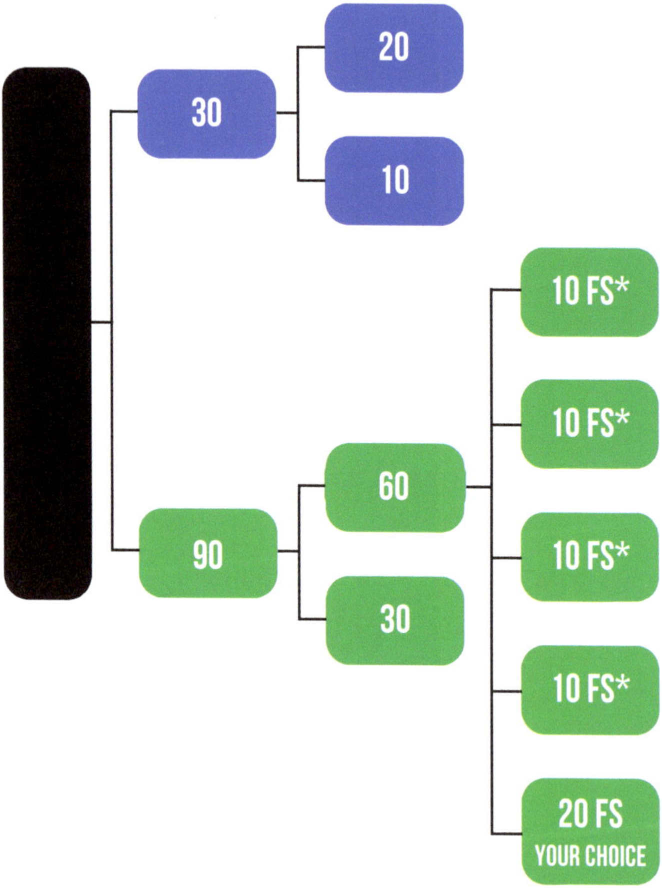

- 30
  - 20
  - 10
- 90
  - 60
    - 10 FS*
    - 10 FS*
    - 10 FS*
    - 10 FS*
    - 20 FS **YOUR CHOICE**
  - 30

SURGICAL SPECIALTIES (EXCLUDING GENERAL SURGERY)

- Cardiothoracic
- Genitourinary
- Neurology
- Obstetrics and Gynecology
- Orthopedic
- Otorhinolaryngology
- Ophthalmology
- Oral Maxillofacial
- Peripheral vascular
- Plastics and reconstructive
- Procurement and transplant

SURGICAL TECHNOLOGY STUDENTS

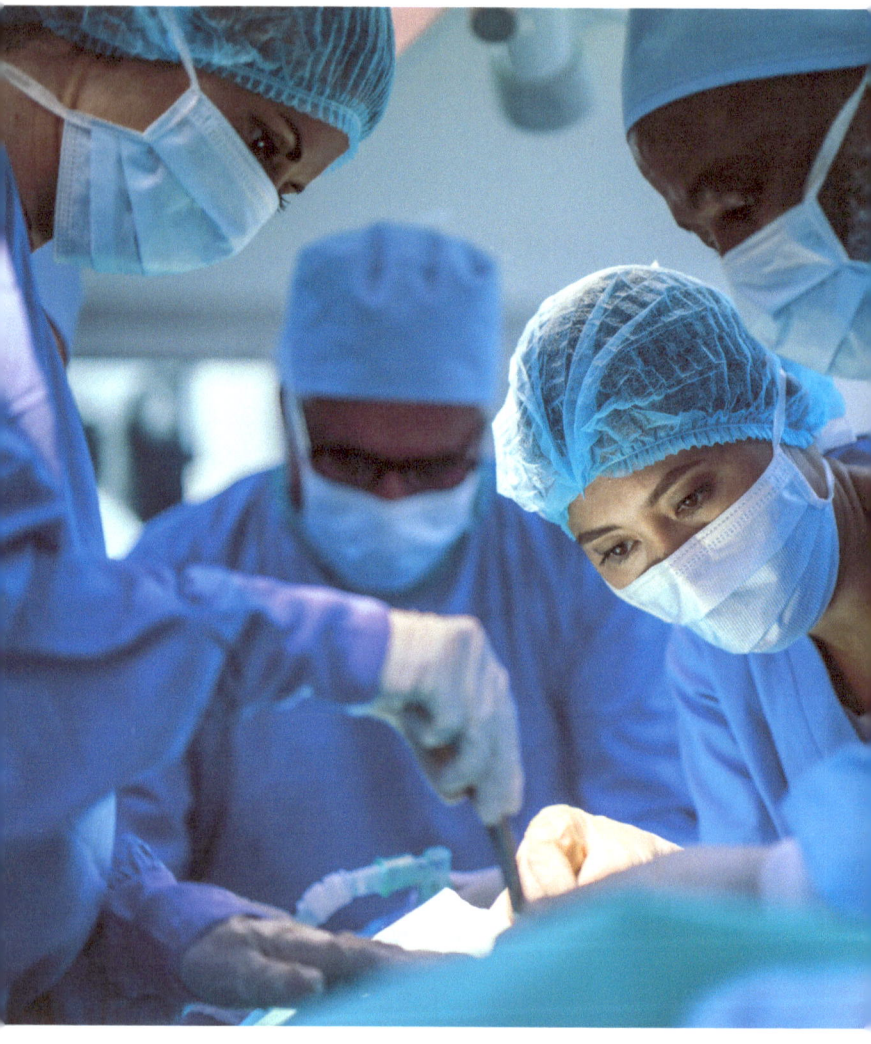

SURGICAL ROTATION CASE AND ROLE DOCUMENTATION

HIT THE GROUND RUNNING

Roles, responsibilities, and definitions in line with AST Core Curriculum 7th Edition

a. **First Scrub Role (FS)**
   To document a case in the FS role, you, as a student, must have performed the following duties during any given surgical procedure with proficiency:

   - ✓ Verify supplies and equipment
   - ✓ Set up the sterile field
   - ✓ Count instruments
   - ✓ Label medication

b. **Second Scrub Role (SS)**

As a student, before you meet all the criteria for the FS role, you may be allowed to actively participate in the surgical procedure from the beginning of the procedure to the end by completing the following in the OR:

- ✓ Assistance with diagnostic endoscopy
- ✓ Assistance with vaginal delivery
- ✓ Cutting suture
- ✓ Providing camera assistance
- ✓ Retracting
- ✓ Sponging
- ✓ Suctioning

c. **Observation Role (O)**
Although the Observation cases cannot be applied to the required 120 case count, they must be recorded in your surgical rotation case log. For the surgical rotation documentation, students can use a cloud-based clinical cases recording tool or a manual log, depending on the program's preference.

d. **Counting cases**
In every procedure, one pathology is counted as one procedure, while more than one case can be counted on a patient. Here are examples of a one pathology case and of counting more than one case on the same patient:

Scenario One (one pathology)
A patient with suspected colon cancer requires a colonoscopy with biopsy; this case of colon cancer screening, which was performed as a diagnostic endoscopic procedure, is counted and documented as one procedure.

Scenario Two (more than one case on the same patient)
A patient requires diagnostic colonoscopy and Esophagogastroduodenoscopy (EGD) procedures. Although they are both endoscopic procedures, they are counted as TWO cases. The colonoscopy is a colon view, while the EGD is the examination of the upper gastrointestinal tract. You will document these as two cases. Your clinical instructor will advise you more on case documentation for full credit.

CASE RECORDING TOOLS:

A cloud -based clinical recording tool or a manual form, Surgical Rotation Documentation (SRD)

Depending on your program, you may be required to record your daily cases using a manual form, Surgical Rotation Documentation (SRD) or using a cloud-based clinical cases recording tool app, for example, Platinum Planner, which automatically tallies your cases electronically. You will receive instructions for either method required by your program. Below is a diagram showing the basic log in screen of a cloud-based clinical recording app:

SURGICAL TECHNOLOGY STUDENTS

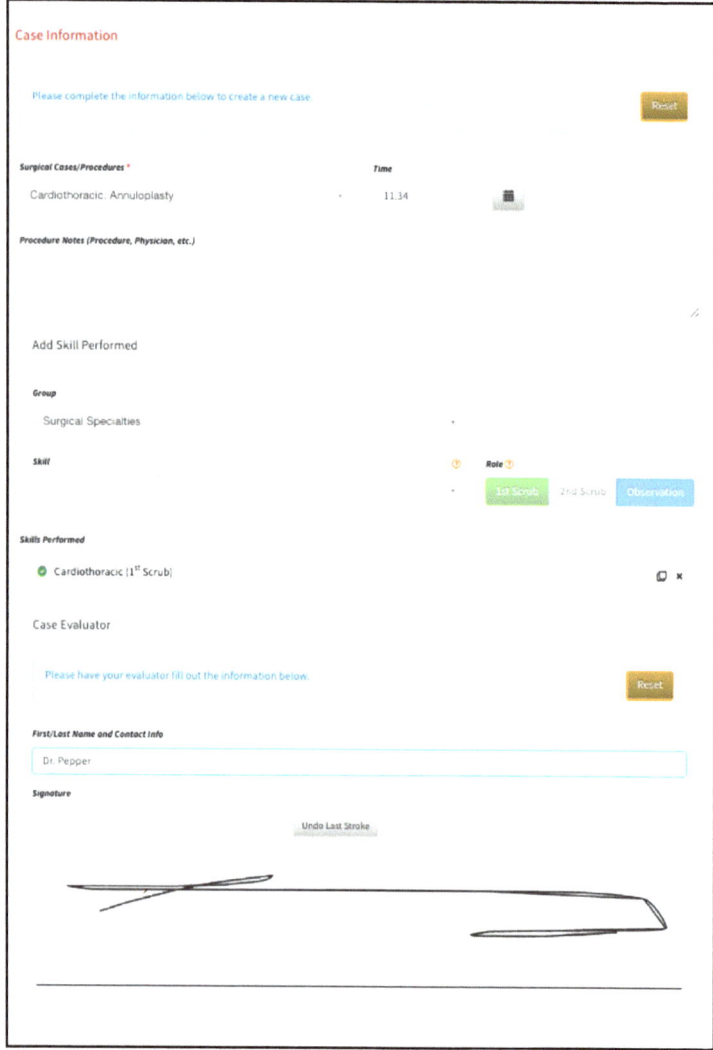

ASSIGNMENTS

A LEARNING AND PRACTICE TOOL: CASE NOTES

Keeping pace with the surgical cases and practicing the step-by-step process of the procedure, using a template to answer set of questions, will help you remember and get familiar with cases as you move along in the operating room. The following information may advance your skills and help you get familiar with surgical procedures in the OR.

Procedure name: Make sure you know the name of the procedure performed.

Definition of procedure: Knowing the meaning of the procedure name will help you understand the procedure better and the reason for the procedure.

The purpose of the procedure: Always find out the reason for a procedure per patient; do not assume the same procedures performed on patients are done for the same reason. One size does not fit all.

The expected outcome of the procedure: Again, the expected outcome of a procedure may be different per patient. Always ask questions per patient and procedure.

Preoperative diagnosis: This is the diagnosis before the surgical procedure.

Discuss the relevant anatomy: The best way to improve your knowledge about the anatomy of the human body is to study and discuss the anatomy in class and with your classmates at any opportunity.

List the general and procedure-specific instruments and equipment that will be needed for the procedure: This will help you to get familiar with instruments and equipment used in the OR for different procedures.

List the basic and procedure-specific supplies that will be needed for the procedure: Surgical packs, Blades, Drapes, Drains, Dressings, and so on.

Types of Sutures and Needles (if applicable): The best way to learn your sutures and needles is to list them by names.

Pharmaceuticals: Always note the medication and the amount used before, during, and after the procedure.

The type of anesthesia used and the reason: Take the opportunity to learn and get familiar with all types of anesthesia.

Patient position during the procedure: This is a very important part of the procedure, as positioning will determine access to the surgical site.

List supplies necessary for positioning: Pay attention to safety aids.

The anatomic perimeters of the prep: Pay attention to proper prepping techniques, especially aseptic techniques. Always prep from clean to dirty to avoid contaminating the clean site. If care is not taken, the patient may end up with an infection.

List the order in which the drapes were applied: Always pay attention to any specific variations and the sequence order of draping.

List the procedural steps: Describe the preparatory and supportive actions of the surgical technologist during each step. This will help you advance your OR anticipating skills faster.

The postoperative diagnosis: Sometimes, the postoperative diagnosis may be different from the preoperative diagnosis because the surgeon may end up performing other surgeries depending on the findings during the procedure.

Describe the immediate postoperative care: Always ask questions of the preceptor or the surgeon when appropriate. You will get more information about postoperative care from the surgeon since the surgeon is the one who recommends care after the procedure. For surgical technologists, care ends in the OR and continues with the Post-Anesthesia Care Unit (PACU) team.

Possible complications: Ask the surgeon about the possible complications after the procedure. There are questions about possible complications in the Surgical Case Report. This will help you prepare your answers for the section when you work on the Surgical Case Report assignments.

Consider all the information you obtained from the surgical team as a tool to use in your assignments and homework, but most of all to utilize in your practice as a surgical technologist.

SURGICAL CASE REPORT

During your clinical rotation, you will be assigned homework assignments pertaining to the procedures in the OR. You will be expected to give details of any surgical procedures that you witnessed or participated in while in a FS, SS or O role. The following are some of the questions you will encounter in your Surgical Case Report assignment:

>The procedure
>
>The surgeon's name
>
>Your preceptor's name
>
>The patient's gender and age
>
>Your role (FS, SS, or O)
>
>Patient allergies, if any

ANATOMY
>A. DESCRIPTION OF AREA OF THE INTENDED SURGICAL INTERVENTION WITH IMMEDIATE ADJOINING STRUCTURES: As you describe the organ or immediate adjoining structures, you will need to provide your source of information. In-text formatting may be necessary for source citations in your paragraph.

B. PATHOLOGY/PURPOSE OF THE SURGERY: Provide the reason(s) for the procedure and ensure to ask the surgeon relevant questions pertaining to each patient. Avoid giving general answers and ensure that all responses are specific to the patient who underwent the procedure.

C. BLOOD SUPPLY TO THE AREA/ORGAN OF THE INTENDED SURGICAL INTERVENTION. You are required to describe the blood supply to the organ and area of the intended surgery. In-text citation may be necessary in your paragraph for source citation.

D. NERVE SUPPLY TO THE AREA/ORGAN OF INTENDED SURGICAL INTERVENTION. You are required to describe the innervation of the organ affected by the surgery. In-text citations may be necessary for this paragraph.

E. PREOPERATIVE DIAGNOSIS. The diagnosis of the patient before the surgery. Always write sentences to answer the questions. Do not give an answer of one word. For example, you may write: "The patient was diagnosed with inguinal hernia."

F. POSTOPERATIVE DIAGNOSIS: Sometimes, the postoperative diagnosis may be different from the preoperative diagnosis because the surgeon may end up performing other surgeries depending on the findings during the procedure. Always write sentences to answer the questions. Do not give an answer of one word. For example, you may write: "The postoperative diagnosis was inguinal hernia which was corrected with mesh placement."

PREOPERATIVE PROCEDURES

PREADMISSION TESTING, IMAGING, AND DIAGNOSTIC STUDIES: Include the preadmission testing that your patient went through before the surgery. Always write sentences to answer the questions. Do not give an answer of one word. For example, you may write: "The surgeon ordered blood work and an ultrasound exam for the patient's heart." Or "The patient had blood drawn and an ultrasound examination of the heart."

EQUIPMENT AND SUPPLIES

A. INSTRUMENTS, SURGICAL PACKS, AND EQUIPMENT. List all instruments, surgical packs and equipment that were used for the surgery.

B. SUTURES. THE SUTURE MATERIAL, THE TYPE OF NEEDLE, AND THE SPECIFIC PART OF THE BODY AND LAYER OF SKIN WHERE IT WAS USED. Always write sentences to answer the questions. Do not give an answer of one word. For example, you may write: "The surgeon preferred to use a nylon suture for the skin. The surgeon used 3 packs of nylon sutures on the toes after the bunionectomy procedure."

C. MEDICATION USED (INCLUDE THE SYRINGE SIZE AND GAUGE OF NEEDLE USED, IF APPLICABLE): List all medications and the amount used during the surgical procedure.

D. TYPE OF ANESTHESIA. If you are not sure of the type of anesthesia used during a procedure, ask the anesthesiologist.

PATIENT POSITIONING
Always provide patient positioning information, including safety considerations and positioning aids. This is crucial!

SURGICAL SITE PREP
Record the solution that was used on the patient's skin, anatomical borders, and all special considerations.

DRAPING
List the material used and the sequence order.

TIMEOUT
Provide information on when and how the timeout was performed. Most importantly, everyone in the room must be quiet, pay close attention to the information given by the circulating nurse, identify themselves, and agree to it before the first incision.

INTRAOPERATIVE PROCEDURES
Provide a detailed description of the procedure, from making the incision to applying the dressing.

POSTOPERATIVE PROCEDURES
This will include the specimen types and handling, PACU care and discharge information from the surgeon, and possible postoperative complications.

CONTINUING EDUCATION ARTICLES

During your third semester of clinical rotation, you will be required to complete Continuing Education articles from the Association of Surgical Technology Journal and answer the provided questions. Your clinical instructor will specify the specific number of articles you need to submit. Your grade will depend on the thoroughness of your answers, the reasoning behind your choices, your enthusiasm, and your understanding of the subject matter.

Using the article as your reference, you must provide in-text citations where necessary and provide a Works Cited page for the articles referenced in your answers. It's important to note that not all surgical technology programs utilize the Continuing Education Article to evaluate students' understanding. Each program may employ varying assessment tools to gauge students' skills, retention, and comprehension during and after their clinical rotation.

BASIC MLA FORMAT

ALWAYS GIVE CREDIT TO YOUR SOURCE OF INFORMATION.

MLA General Guidelines:

Double spaced

1-inch margins on all sides

12 point font size

IN-TEXT CITATIONS AND WORKS CITED PAGES

IN-TEXT CITATIONS

- ✓ Author's last name and page numbers.
- ✓ Website information and page numbers, if applicable.

WORKS CITED PAGE

- ✓ A separate page for the Works Cited page with hanging indents.
- ✓ List of sources alphabetized by the author's surname.
- ✓ Left-aligned with hanging indents.
- ✓ Double-spaced.
- ✓ 1-inch margins.

If your program does not use MLA formatting, you will be provided with the formatting style your program prefers. Please visit https://owl.purdue.edu for step-by-step guides and examples of all formatting styles.

ARE YOU READY FOR THE CLINICAL ROTATION?

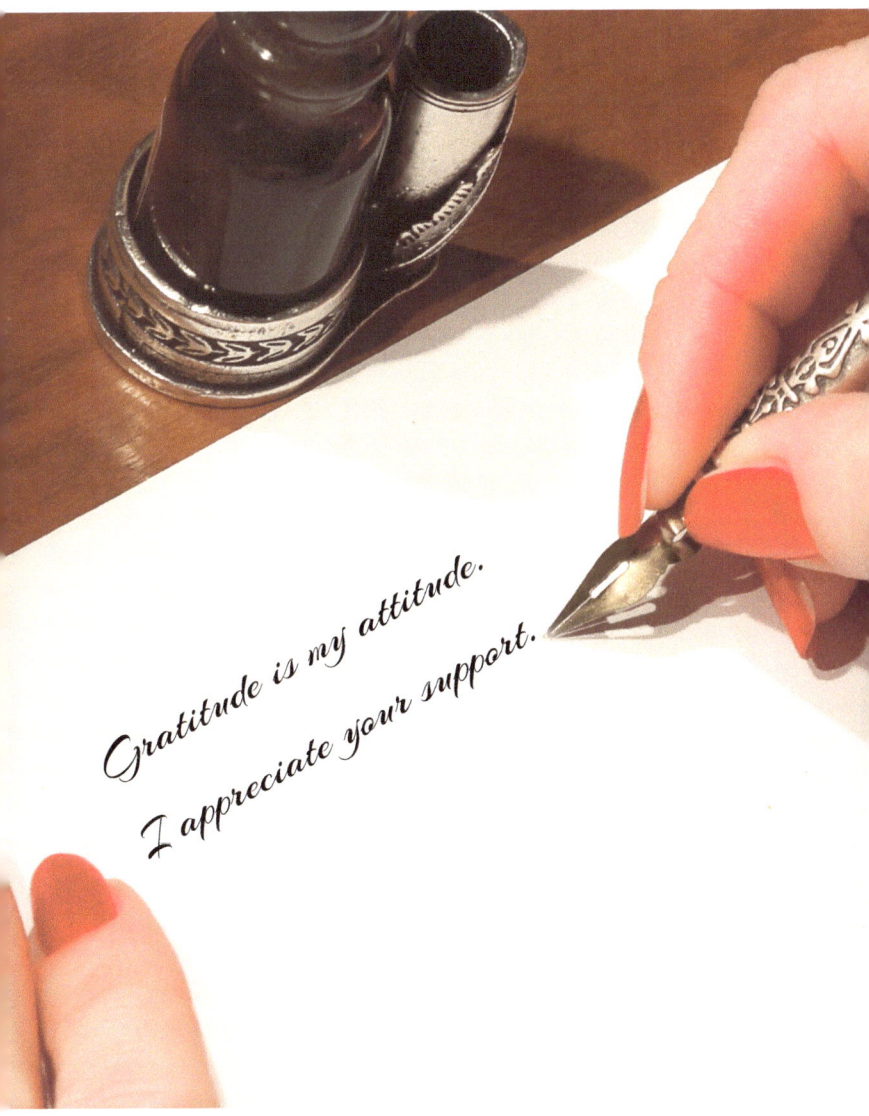

SURGICAL TECHNOLOGY STUDENTS

MANUAL SURGICAL CASE RECORDING TOOL
GENERAL SURGERY

NO.	DATE	PROCEDURE	FIRST SCRUB	SECOND SCRUB
1.				
2				
3.				
4.				
5.				
6.				
7.				
8.				
9.				
10.				
11.				
12.				
13.				
14.				
15.				
16.				
17.				
18.				
19.				
20.				
21.				
22.				
23.				
24.				
25.				
26.				
26.				
28.				
29.				
30.				

OBSERVATION ROLE
(NOT APPLIED TO REQUIRED CASE COUNT)

NO.	DATE	SPECIALTY	PROCEDURE
1.			
2			
3.			
4.			
5.			
6.			
7.			
8.			
9.			
10.			
11.			
12.			
13.			
14.			
15.			
16.			
17.			
18.			
19.			
20.			
21.			
22.			
23.			
24.			
25.			
26.			
26.			
28.			
29.			
30.			

SURGICAL TECHNOLOGY STUDENTS

CARDIOTHORACIC

NO.	DATE	PROCEDURE	FIRST SCRUB	SECOND SCRUB
1.				
2				
3.				
4.				
5.				
6.				
7.				
8.				
9.				
10.				
11.				
12.				
13.				
14.				
15.				

GENITOURINARY

NO.	DATE	PROCEDURE	FIRST SCRUB	SECOND SCRUB
1.				
2				
3.				
4.				
5.				
6.				
7.				
8.				
9.				
10.				
11.				
12.				
13.				
14.				
15.				

NEUROLOGY

NO.	DATE	PROCEDURE	FIRST SCRUB	SECOND SCRUB
1.				
2				
3.				
4.				
5.				
6.				
7.				
8.				
9.				
10.				
11.				
12.				
13.				
14.				
15.				

OBSTETRICS AND GYNECOLOGY

NO.	DATE	PROCEDURE	FIRST SCRUB	SECOND SCRUB
1.				
2				
3.				
4.				
5.				
6.				
7.				
8.				
9.				
10.				
11.				
12.				
13.				
14.				
15.				

ORTHOPEDIC

NO.	DATE	PROCEDURE	FIRST SCRUB	SECOND SCRUB
1.				
2				
3.				
4.				
5.				
6.				
7.				
8.				
9.				
10.				
11.				
12.				
13.				
14.				
15.				

OTORHINOLARYNGOLOGY

NO.	DATE	PROCEDURE	FIRST SCRUB	SECOND SCRUB
1.				
2				
3.				
4.				
5.				
6.				
7.				
8.				
9.				
10.				
11.				
12.				
13.				
14.				
15.				

ARE YOU READY FOR THE CLINICAL ROTATION?

OPHTHALMOLOGY

NO.	DATE	PROCEDURE	FIRST SCRUB	SECOND SCRUB
1.				
2				
3.				
4.				
5.				
6.				
7.				
8.				
9.				
10.				
11.				
12.				
13.				
14.				
15.				

ORAL MAXILLOFACIAL

NO.	DATE	PROCEDURE	FIRST SCRUB	SECOND SCRUB
1.				
2				
3.				
4.				
5.				
6.				
7.				
8.				
9.				
10.				
11.				
12.				
13.				
14.				
15.				

PERIPHERAL VASCULAR

NO.	DATE	PROCEDURE	FIRST SCRUB	SECOND SCRUB
1.				
2				
3.				
4.				
5.				
6.				
7.				
8.				
9.				
10.				
11.				
12.				
13.				
14.				
15.				

PLASTIC AND RECONSTRUCTIVE

NO.	DATE	PROCEDURE	FIRST SCRUB	SECOND SCRUB
1.				
2				
3.				
4.				
5.				
6.				
7.				
8.				
9.				
10.				
11.				
12.				
13.				
14.				
15.				

PROCUREMENT AND TRANSPLANT

NO.	DATE	PROCEDURE	FIRST SCRUB	SECOND SCRUB
1.				
2				
3.				
4.				
5.				
6.				
7.				
8.				
9.				
10.				
11.				
12.				
13.				
14.				
15.				

ENDOSCOPY

NO.	DATE	PROCEDURE	SECOND SCRUB
1.			
2			
3.			
4.			
5.			
6.			
7.			
8.			
9.			
10.			
11.			
12.			
13.			
14.			
15.			

SURGICAL TECHNOLOGY STUDENTS

NOTES

NOTES

SURGICAL TECHNOLOGY STUDENTS

NOTES

ARE YOU READY FOR THE CLINICAL ROTATION?

NOTES

ABOUT THE AUTHOR

Francisca Soetan, EdD, CST, is a respected faculty member at Kingsborough Community College, City University of New York, specializing in Allied Health, Mental Health, and Human Services.

With over 18 years of experience as a surgical technologist in Brooklyn hospitals and surgical centers, she brings a wealth of practical knowledge to her students. Her passion lies in teaching surgical technology, a dream she is living out at Kingsborough. Author of Surgical Technology Students - Are You Ready for The Clinical Rotation? Clinical Rotation Guide for The Surgical Technology Student, Soetan is committed to guiding aspiring surgical technologists on their educational journey.

www.ingramcontent.com/pod-product-compliance
Lightning Source LLC
LaVergne TN
LVHW070433080526
838201LV00129B/264